The Ultimate Truth, Knowledge & Wisdom

notionpress.com

The Ultimate Truth, Knowledge & Wisdom

Sanjay Goel

notionpress.com

Notion Press

Old No. 38, New No. 6

McNichols Road, Chetpet

Chennai - 600 031

First Published by Notion Press 2015

ISBN 978-93-5206-586-8

Contents

PREFACE

This book discusses the most fundamental aspects of life such as the purpose of our existence, human nature and the effect of thinking and philosophy on our psychological and physical health. It goes on to detail the various methods of meditation and their effect on physical health as well as on the ultimate quest to reach the Supreme.

It deals with death, the soul, ancient Vedic philosophy, non-violence, the effect of philosophy on relationships and achievements in life, dreams and detachment.

It guides a person on how to lead a balanced life and attain the ultimate purpose of human existence, which is peace and bliss. It explains that the human mind is always disturbed, restless and wandering in the past, present and future. Due to ignorance and attachments, there is the false belief that these materialistic objects would give more satisfaction and happiness than at present or more than what one already has. The more he obtains these objects, the more man's desires increase, like adding fuel to fire and he is always torn between the dualities of life–death, happiness–sorrow, gain–loss, good–evil and so on.

Only that person who understands that there is nothing to achieve or lose in this world can rise above these dualities, as the two sides of dualities like life–death, happiness–sorrow, gain–loss, good–evil and so on shall always be equal to each other, and one cannot exist without an equal amount of the other. The person who understands the above truth knows that he is neither living nor dead, neither happy nor unhappy, neither good nor evil and so on. He rises above these dualities, does all his duties in life without any desire or aversion and attains ultimate peace and bliss.

The Three Personalities

No two human beings are exactly similar. Every human being is unique in his nature, and his personality depends upon many factors including his background, education, place of origin, residence, religion, friends' circle, economic condition and so on. However, the natures of human beings can be broadly classified into three categories:

The first category of persons is those who think positively about themselves. They think that they are immortal, everything, rich, powerful, influential, creator, preserver and destroyer of this Universe, masters, wise, handsome/beautiful, superior to others and so on. Such category of persons base their thinking on the philosophy that they are not this body but an indestructible soul, this Universe is a small part of their mind and hence they are its creators, preservers and destroyers. They also think they are superior to other human beings as they are more influential, educated, rich and powerful than others and so on.

Such category of persons are very ambitious, swift in their actions, hardworking, set very high aims in life, and are short–tempered, extremely competitive, move in high circles and look down upon other fellow human beings as inferior.

Such type of persons suffer from lifestyle disorders such as anxiety, acidity, insomnia, superiority complex, over working, weak digestion, bad temper and so on. They are unable to control their anger and cannot tolerate even the slightest offence or mistake of other people. Gradually, such people develop more serious health and psychological problems and either have to seek medical help or abandon their above mentioned philosophy and move on to other categories mentioned below.

The second category of persons is those who think negatively about themselves. They think that they are destructible, nothing, weak, insignificant, illusory, uneducated, inferior, ugly, diseased, subordinates and so on.

Such persons base their thinking on the philosophy that they are mortal and would die one day. They think that they are only a speck of dust in this endless Universe and they were not there before their birth, would not be there after their death and hence in the present or in between also they are merely an illusion. They also think that one day everything would end and would be reduced to dust and is henceforth totally meaningless. They also think they are extremely weak, powerless, uneducated, ugly, servants and so on.

Such type of people suffer from lifestyle disorders such as depression, panic attacks, sadism, pessimism, lack of interest, lethargy, low productivity, low self esteem, substance abuse, insomnia, over forgiveness, loneliness, poverty and so on.

Gradually, the problems faced by such people get worse and they develop more serious health and psychological problems and are forced to seek medical help or abandon their above mentioned philosophy and move on to the other categories.

The third category of persons is those who think neither positively nor negatively about themselves and are neutral. They think that they are neither mortal nor immortal, neither everything nor nothing, neither good nor evil, neither strong nor weak, neither rich nor poor and so on.

Such type of persons base their thinking on the philosophy that one side of the dualities like life–death, happiness–sorrow, mortal–immortal, good–evil, light–darkness, night–day and so on shall always be equal to other and one cannot exist without an equal amount of the other, and therefore there is nothing to achieve or lose in this world and no situation in life is better than the other.

Persons of this type lead a balanced, healthy and peaceful life. They are not easily disturbed by the dualities or ups and downs in life. While the other two categories of people are restless like waves or a pendulum and keep on moving from one category to another, this type of people are peaceful like an ocean. A person of this type does all his duties in life without any desire or hatred as he understands that there is nothing to achieve or lose in this world and hence become a Karma Yogi and attains a state of perfect peace or bliss.

Purpose of Life

The real purpose of life is to understand that there is no purpose. In other words, there is purpose in no purpose and no purpose in purpose. If you ask any human being on this earth about the purpose of his life, the most likely answer would be to attain and enjoy materialistic pleasures like wealth, education, family, friends, fame, health and so on.

If we first look at wealth, then we shall find that the richest people on this earth have not been able to find any happiness in their wealth beyond provision of basic necessities of life. Therefore it is no wonder that many of the richest people have taken to philanthropy or giving up their wealth for the welfare of other people in order to find more meaning in life.

Similarly, if we look at educational qualifications, then also we find that education these days only teaches about the materialistic world or the art of making money, and does not teach you anything about the methods of obtaining peace and contentment. No wonder, even medical professionals these days abuse drugs in order to relax.

If we look at large families, then also we find that having a family does not guarantee you any peace. Violent clashes among family members over petty issues are quite common. The larger the family, more are the disputes.

As far as friends are concerned, they are also of not much use beyond a certain level. Moreover, if you keep bad company, then instead of finding happiness, you will get into more trouble in life. The greater the number of friends one has, the greater are his enemies. Moreover, most of your enemies today were your friends at some point of time and vice versa.

If we look at fame and popularity, then also we find that famous people are not very happy in their lives and they have frequent quarrels with photographers and journalists over intrusion into their privacy. Some of the most famous people on this earth have died unnatural deaths due to drug overdose, alcohol, accidents and murders, and they blamed their popularity for most of their miseries in life.

If we look at health, then also we find that having good health is no guarantee for peace and contentment. People only think about the importance of good health when they are ill, otherwise nobody bothers about it. Many people who are physically healthy are mentally disturbed, and it is not surprising that most of the criminals in jail enjoy good health as an ill person is not in a position to commit crime.

People run after materialistic pleasure under the false impression that it will provide them with peace and happiness in life, but the more they try to achieve them, the more their desire increases, like adding fuel to fire, and in the end instead of giving them peace, these materialistic pleasures make them more disturbed. Everybody in this world is trying to deceive the other person by only trying to show his positive side and by hiding the negative side. For example, a person will only show his photograph when he is smiling or enjoying but never when he is crying or quarrelling with somebody. It is human nature to ape other persons and when a person sees the positive side of another person, he falsely believes that the other person is happier than himself without understanding his negative side, and tries to ape him thinking that the grass is greener on the other side. This leads to endless competition, disturbance and rat race as everybody is in a hurry to outsmart the other person. In the end they end up more disturbed and discontented and forget that one day even their own body for which they are taking so much effort would deceive them and would be reduced to dust or ashes.

There are certain people who take up philanthropy or the welfare of other living beings in order to find more meaning and peace in life, but they are also not very successful as the word 'welfare' is subjective, and its meaning may differ from person to person. For example giving alms to a beggar or feeding stray dogs, monkeys and other animals may be an act of philanthropy or welfare from your point of view, but a big nuisance from the point of view of other people and the law of the land. Also, the act of giving alms will make that person dependent upon you, and he would lose his motivation to work hard in life, and you may end up doing more harm to him than any good. Similar is the case with all other human activities. Therefore, people looking for peace in philanthropy or welfare of other living beings are also not very successful.

There are certain people who try to go deeper into the purpose of life and try to look up answers in various religious scriptures and philosophy, but there also they may not be very successful as they may find conflicting views in them. For example, on the one hand ancient Vedic philosophy says that if you do good Karma you go to heaven, and if you do bad Karma you go to hell, while on the other hand it says that not even a blade of grass can move without the will of God. Now the question is that if everything is done by God, then why should anybody go to heaven or hell, and if everything depends upon our Karma, then how is God powerful or relevant? Also, at certain places it says that heaven and hell are also an illusion like this Universe and have been created only to encourage people to move towards the right path of restraining their senses, achieving detachment and liberation or peace, which leaves a person even more confused. However, regarding the ultimate purpose of life, it is absolutely clear that liberation or freedom from endless dualities and the cycle of life–death, happiness–sorrow, gain–loss, heat–cold and so on, and attaining eternal peace and bliss, is the ultimate purpose of life. Many methods have been suggested to attain the above objective, such as Raja Yoga, Gyan Yoga, Bhakti Yoga and Karma Yoga, which are not easy to understand without the guidance of an able Guru, and it is extremely difficult to find such a Guru, as such people do not openly display their knowledge, but stay alone, maintain silence and don't have any desire in life. Moreover, the methods stated above are conflicting to each other and a person may find it difficult to choose one over the other.

Now the final question is as to what is the purpose of life? The answer is that understanding that there is no purpose is the real purpose of life. In other words, there is no purpose in purpose and there is purpose in no purpose. The earth keeps on revolving around the Sun, what is the purpose? Or, you throw a stone into space, which will keep on moving endlessly because of zero resistance; what is the purpose? Or there might be endless planets like the earth containing endless life forms in the Universe, what is the purpose? Or, you consider yourself as living, and non-living things as dead, but they are as much living as you are and you are as much dead as them, what is the purpose? Or you might have taken endless births and died an endless number of times by now, what is the purpose?

The answer to all these questions is that there is no purpose, or that there is purpose in no purpose, and no purpose in purpose. We human beings consider ourselves to be living and more intelligent than other life forms and non-living things, but fail to see that non-living things are as much living as we are, and we are as much dead as they are. Every moment millions of living cells of our body die and are replaced by new ones, and similarly every moment billions of so called non-living things are converting themselves into living cells and organisms. This means that every moment we are living as well as dying, and non-living things are also dying and living every moment like us. We consider ourselves to be more intelligent and evolved, but the so called non-living things might be equally or more evolved than us, that is, they might have already realized or experienced that there is purpose in no purpose, and no purpose in purpose. Only that person can realize this ultimate truth in life who understands that the two sides of dualities like life–death, happiness–sorrow, good–evil, and gain–loss shall always be equal to each other, and one cannot exist without an equal amount of the other, and therefore there is nothing to achieve or lose in this world. Once a person understands the above truth, he rises above these dualities and realizes his ultimate purpose, peace and bliss.

Qualities of A Good Leader

There are many qualities of a good leader and all of these can be classified under three main categories which are mention below:

1. Do for others what you expect them to do for you.
2. Conquer your own mind and senses before you attempt to conquer the hearts and minds of others.
3. Take all decisions with a detached mind and be indifferent to the results.

Now as far as the first quality is concerned, it is necessary that you set an example to your followers, employees and children through actions and not words. It is a natural tendency of people to follow or ape their leaders, teachers, employers and parents as they consider them to be their role models. If you want your followers to work hard, you will first have to set an example before them with your hard work, and mere plain advice or talks will not work. Similarly, if you want your employees, followers & children to be honest, forgiving, devoted and truthful, then you will first have to show them the path with your own honesty, forgiveness, devotion and truthfulness.

If you want them to follow you and sacrifice anything for you, then you will first have to allow them to lead and make similar sacrifices for them. If you just keep on verbally advising them without yourself following the advice, they will soon start ignoring you and you will lose all respect.

Now, as far as the second quality is considered, it is necessary that a leader be in firm control of his mind, senses and desires before he leads others. A person, who conquers his own self, can conquer the entire world, and a person who is a slave of his own mind and senses, cannot lead anybody. A person who is always busy in satisfying his senses through various entertainment programs in television/internet or intoxicates himself through liquor/drugs, or runs too much after luxuries in life such as expensive cars, aircrafts, women, expensive hotels, food etc. or socializes too much, soon drowns in these unproductive activities and is not able to concentrate upon his work and becomes out of touch with various developments. Such a person is outsmarted by his competitors and rivals. The employees, followers and children of such a person also ape him and become like him. In the end all of them are ruined and try to put the blame on each other for their downfall. On the contrary, a person who is dedicated and also devotes some of his time to meditation, becomes very sharp and will soon be able to outsmart his rivals. The followers of such a person also praise and follow him, respecting his deep knowledge and hold on the subject and they all progress together.

Now, the third important quality of a leader is that he should take all decisions with a detached mind and be indifferent to results. A person, who is attached, is always disturbed by the ups and downs of life such as profit–loss, happiness–sorrow and so on. Such a person's mind gets clouded with these unproductive emotions which leads him to a wrong decision. Most of the wrong decisions taken by a person are when he is extremely angry or excited. This fact can be verified from most of the criminals in jail who blame their anger or over excitement for their crimes and the wrong steps taken by them in life. Also, to control these extreme emotions, people take to intoxication through liquor/drugs/medical prescriptions, so that their mind gets diverted for some time. Soon they become dependent upon such intoxicating substances and are unable to concentrate upon their work, which leads to their downfall. Seeing such leaders running away from truth or work through these intoxicants, the employees and followers also follow them, and all of them together move towards failure. On the contrary a person who takes all decisions with a calm, peaceful and composed mind always takes the right decision. Such a person does not care about the end results and only thinks about social welfare. Such a person soon rises to dizzying heights and gains the respect of everybody. But the biggest problem is how to achieve this state of mind where the person is detached and indifferent to the results, without which it is not possible to attain even the other two qualities mentioned above.

The answer is that he can achieve the above state when he understands that there is nothing to achieve or lose in this world, as the two sides of the dualities like profit–gain, good–evil, life–death, negative–positive and so on shall always be equal to each other, and one cannot exist without an equal amount of the other. As soon as a person realizes the above truth, he becomes detached and indifferent to all his actions in life, conquers this mind and senses, and starts thinking about the welfare of other people as his false ego gets shattered. Such a person gains all the three qualities of a leader as stated above and attains ultimate peace and bliss in life.

Life and Death

Like everything else in this Universe, we are neither living nor dead. But when time/space separates out the dualities within us which were in equal proportion within is, then we start experiencing both life and death in equal proportions. In 'Garuda Purana', Lord Vishnu while imparting knowledge to Garuda (chapter 11, verse 3) states that "A person who has taken birth is bound to die and a person who has died is bound to be reborn". Life and Death in a person can be compared to the state of being awake and asleep. The only difference between death and sleep is that when a person is reborn he has no memory of the past, and is born with a new body. In other words, if you sleep at night and wake up in the morning without any memory of the past and with a new body, then that sleep is nothing but your Death.

Now, the question is whether the person who has taken birth after his death is a new person or the same old one? The answer is, when you sleep at night and get up in the morning without a past memory and with a new body, you are neither the same person nor a new one. In other words, though your consciousness is the same, you have no memory of the past and have a new body. In the case of death also, the answer is the same; when you are reborn, neither are you the same person nor a new person. In other words you are neither mortal nor immortal.

Now, the question is, why do we die? The answer is that after working for a certain period of time, both your body and mind wear out and become useless. Your body is unable to work anymore and your mind also gets saturated with memories and unable to hold anymore. Therefore, nature takes away the old worn out body and provides you with a new one. It is like when you eat your food, once the body digests it and extracts nutrients from it, it throws out the waste product. Similarly, when you have lived your life, nature extracts your experiences and Karmas from your old body and provides them to you in the form of a new body and nature (Sanskar). Your past experiences and Karmas are not lost but are passed on. This is how life has evolved from a microbe to the present diversity. Ancient Vedic philosophy also states that only after millions of births do you get the human body. There is a very interesting recent scientific experiment in which a mouse was exposed to an electric shock associated with certain experience or memory like smell, so that whenever the mouse is exposed to that particular memory/experience it develops a fear of it. It was noticed that even though its off springs were not exposed to similar electric shocks, they naturally had the fear of that particular experience/memory/smell, as the mouse had biologically transferred that experience to its off springs. Similarly, our past experiences and Karmas are passed on to us in the form of a new body and nature (Sanskar). The new body is neither the same person nor a different one. Now, the question is why does time/space separate the dualities like life–death within us, when they were earlier in a state of perfect harmony? The answer is that it was because of your own desire to experience something new that the dualities were separated out within you. Earlier when you were neither living nor dead, you were in a state of perfect peace and harmony like a still ocean or water, but when the time/space separated out the dualities within you because of your desire, you became disturbed like a wave. When the wave goes up, it is your life and when the wave goes down, it is your death. It is a continuous process.

Now, the final question is how can we became still again and attain our earlier state of Peace & Harmony? The answer is, by conquering your endless desires and attaining a state of indifference towards all situations in life. This can be done when you understand that desires can never be fulfilled and trying to satisfy them is like running after a mirage. The more you try to satisfy them, the more will they increase. You can become indifferent by understanding that there is nothing to achieve or lose in this world, as one side of the duality such as life–death, happiness–sorrow, good–evil, day–night and so on, shall always be equal to each other, and one cannot exist without an equal amount of the other. The person who understands the above truth gradually slows down and attains his original perfect state of peace and bliss.

Ramayana and Mahabharata of Life

Your life is one big battle. There is a constant struggle in your life which has been clearly reflected in the Ramayana and the Mahabharata. We keep on blaming our stars, health, friends, family members, colleagues, neighbors, parents, business associates and so on for the various troubles in our lives, but forget that our biggest enemy or Ravana who is responsible for all our troubles is our own mind only.

If we compare our lives to the Ramayana then we are Rama and our three brothers Lakshmana, Bharat and Shatrughna are represented by our devotion, sacrifice and compassion. Hanuman is our strength, Vibhishana is love, Dasharatha is truth, Angad is forgiveness, Jambavana is honesty, Jatayu is charity, Sage Vashishta is knowledge, Sugreeva is sincerity, Nala is patience and Neel is purity. Our army or Vanarsena is detachment. Our greatest enemy Ravana is our mind, his ten heads are our ten senses, Soorpanakha is lust, Meghanada is falsehood and Kumbhkarna is ignorance. Ravana's army is the various objects of senses or desire. Our enemy wants to capture us in the prison of our endless desires.

Similarly, if we compare our lives with Mahabharata, then we are Lord Krishna, while Pandavas, that is, Yudhishtira, Bheema, Arjuna, Nakula and Sahdev are represented by our virtue, physical strength, sacrifice, love and compassion respectively. Abhimanyu is charity, Satyaki is truth, and the five sons of Draupadi are forgiveness, honesty, simplicity, purity and sincerity. Virat is equanimity, Sage Vyas is Knowledge and Drupad is patience. Our army is detachment. Our biggest enemy Duryodhana is our mind and Bheeshma, Drona, Kripa, Karna, Dushasana, Ashwatthama, Shalya, Shakuni, Bhoorisharava and Bhagdutt are our ten senses, Dhratrashtra is ignorance and Alambush is falsehood. The army of our enemy consists of various objects of senses or desire. Again, our enemy wants to capture us in the prison of endless desires and ignorance.

Our enemy is very powerful and attacks us from three directions simultaneously. The first is through its army of various objects of senses or desire. The said army can only be defeated through our army of detachment. We can become detached only if we understand that our desires are endless and the entire objects of senses in this world are not sufficient to satisfy even one person. The more we try to satisfy our desires, the more they increase like adding fuel to fire.

The second attack is from our ten senses which are trying to capture us and take us out of this body towards various objects of senses and endless desires. They can only be defeated if we attack them through our army of ten great warriors which are truth, forgiveness, honesty, simplicity, charity, purity, sincerity, compassion, equanimity and patience. These ten warriors will force our ten senses to surrender and stop wandering outside in the world of various objects of senses and desires, and move inwards.

The third and the most formidable attack is from our greatest enemy which is our mind. This mind is always restlessly moving in the past or future for satisfying itself with various objects of senses or desires, under the false impression that realization of these desires or objects would give it more satisfaction than at present. The more it realizes these desires, the more restless it becomes. The only way to defeat this enemy is through the weapon or 'Brahmastra' of indifference.

You can attain this state of indifference if you understand that there is nothing to achieve or lose in this world, as one side of the duality like life–death, happiness–sorrow, good–evil, night–day and so on shall always be equal to the other and one cannot exist without an equal amount of the other. In other words, no situation in life is better or worse than the other. The moment you realize the above truth, you will become indifferent to all situations in life, and this weapon of indifference will defeat your greatest enemy which is your restless mind. The moment you defeat it you will stop moving up and down endlessly like a wave between dualities of life–death, happiness–sorrow, gain–loss and so on, and attain the state of perfect peace and bliss.

Seed of the Universe

You are the seed of this Universe. Earlier you were like a seed where all dualities like life–death, happiness–sorrow, good–evil, day–night, and so on, which are always equal to each other were in perfect harmony within you. In other words you were neither living nor dead, neither happy nor unhappy, neither good nor evil and so on, and were in a state of perfect peace or bliss. Later on, this seed or you received the nourishment of the water of desire. Once it got this nourishment in the form of desire, it grew with a big bang into a massive and endless tree which is known as this Universe. Your consciousness is the root of this tree, your mind is the main stem/trunk, the five basic elements (i.e. Earth, Water, Fire, Air, Sky) are its five main branches, your ten senses (i.e. eyes, ears, nose, tongue, skin, voice, legs, hands, anus, genitals) are the ten sub-branches of the tree. The five objects of senses i.e. smell, taste, touch, form and sound are the leaves of this tree. Your Karmas are the manure for this tree, and it bears the beautiful flowers of happiness and the bitter fruits of pain. This tree of Universe is within you and you are within this Universe like a seed.

When you were the seed, all the dualities were in perfect harmony within you, and you experienced perfect peace or bliss. But when you grew into this massive tree, the said dualities were separated within you by time/space, and you started experiencing both life–death, happiness–sorrow, profit–loss and so on in equal proportions and became extremely restless like waves which keep on going up and down, or the pendulum of a clock which keeps on moving from side to side. Your mind is endlessly wandering in the past, present and future for achieving certain goals in life which you falsely believe will give you more satisfaction and happiness than the present. All the time you are chasing that mirage and never are you able to achieve your endless desires and goals.

Now, the question is how to again achieve that state of perfect peace and bliss, that is, how to become that seed again? The answer is–first of all stop feeding this tree with the water of endless desires.

This can be done by understanding that all the objects of senses in this world are not sufficient to satisfy even one person. The more you try to enjoy these objects the more your desire will increase like adding fuel to fire. Once, you become detached from the objects of senses, you will find that this tree has become dry and weak. Once it has weakened, cut this tree with the axe of indifference. You can become indifferent if you understand that there is nothing to achieve or lose in this world, as the two sides of the dualities will always be equal to each other. The more you will try to run after profit, the more loss you will suffer, the more you try to run after happiness, the more sorrow you will get, and so on.

You should sit down and quietly meditate for at least half an hour every day, reminding yourself at regular intervals that there is nothing to achieve or lose in this world, as your gains and losses shall always be equal in all situations of life. You will find that after meditating for some time, your mind has become more peaceful and has stopped wandering in the past or future. Your sight will get fixed in between your eyebrows. Instead of looking outside, your vision will turn inwards. You will start experiencing certain divine emotions, beauty and objects which are beyond words. Time will slow down and you will experience that everything around you including your thoughts are moving in slow motion. Slowly and steadily, with practice you will conquer the time/space which have separated the two dualities, and become the seed again with a big crunch and attain Samadhi/Nirvana, which is the state of perfect peace or bliss, which is your true self.

Non-Violence

Non-violence is regarded as the highest virtue by ancient Vedic, Jain and Buddhist philosophy. Other religions have also taught the importance of non-violence. Mahatma Gandhi and several other world leaders also practiced and preached the virtues of non-violence. According to Vedic philosophy, non-violence means not harming any living being through actions, words or mind. Violence is of two types, one is voluntary and the other is involuntary. Here violence only refers to voluntary or pre-planned violence and not to the involuntary or essential violence. Involuntary or essential violence is happening all the time and we have no control over it. For example our bodies are killing fields and our immune system is a killing machine. Every moment millions of foreign microbes, viruses and bacteria enter our body through air, water and food, and if our immune system does not identify and kill these harmful organisms, we will not survive even for a moment. Other examples of involuntary violence include eating plant based or complete vegan diet which is devoid of all animal products. In such a diet, even though pain is not visible to us but still there is a possibility that it is there as we are consuming grains, seeds, pulses, roots etc. which are living foods. There are innumerable other examples like walking, tilling of land, eating and so on and we cannot even breathe or move even a finger without causing violence to some or the other organism. There is another category of involuntary or essential violence which is caused to prevent a greater violence or greater harm to the society, like arrests made by the police, punishment given by the judges, enemies killed by the soldiers or painful medical operations carried out by the doctors. Such type of violence, if not done, would result in a much greater violence to the society. The said category of involuntary or essential violence is not violence, and the person indulging in it does not in any way morally or physically incur any repercussions or adverse consequences for his acts. Even Lord Krishna in Bhagvad Gita taught Arjuna to fight for the righteous battle when he refused to fight against his own teachers and relatives for fear of violence. Lord Krishna told Arjuna that it is his duty as a soldier to fight a righteous battle and running away from it would amount to cowardice, and he would lose his self respect and also incur sin for such cowardice. Similarly, law also punishes the public servants like police officers, judges, and army personnel who refuse to do their duties involving violence out is fear or cowardice, and rewards those who perform their duties involving violence efficiently. Therefore both religion and law do not regard involuntary or essential violence as violence or wrong.

As far as voluntary or non-essential violence is concerned, it is regarded as sin by both religion as well as the law of the land. While religion states that the sinner would be punished by God or nature for his act, law of the land awards punishments through courts of justice. It is our common experience that a person reaps what he sows or whatever a person does comes back to him in some or the other form. The examples of voluntary violence include killing or torturing innocent human beings and animals for illegal personal gain or pleasure.

Now, most of the human beings would agree that causing voluntary violence without justification is wrong.

But the problem is that no person on this earth can remain without work even for a moment, and no human activity can be carried out without violence. Every human activity like agriculture, industry, justice, administration, walking, eating, drinking, and breathing involves some or the other kind of violence, and it has both voluntary as well as involuntary violence. In the Gita Lord Krishna tells Arjuna that every human activity or Karma has some vice or negative aspect (Dosha), just like fire that is always surrounded or accompanied by smoke (chapter 18, verse 47). For example, while growing the crops, a farmer not only kills various organisms involuntarily while tilling the land, but also voluntarily causes harm to them while protecting his crops from insects and other animals. Similar is the case for every other human activity. Now, the question then is how will human beings survive without violence? The answer is given in the Gita by Lord Krishna that when a person does any Karma or activity without any attachment or expectation of results, his Karma or activity becomes "akarma" or non-activity. In other words even while performing his duties, he does not incur any good or bad fruits of action (chapter 5, verse 9), and such a person is ultimately liberated or attains peace and bliss.

Now, the final question is, why should a person be detached or do his duties without any expectation of results, when every person in this world works only for some reward or motive? The answer is, because there is nothing to achieve or lose in this world as one side of dualities like good–evil, life–death, happiness–sorrow, gain–loss and so on shall always be equal to the other, and one cannot exist without an equal amount of the other. A person who understands the above truth rises above these dualities and also realizes that all human acts have equal amount of good–evil, gain–loss, negative–positive and so on and becomes detached from them and their results. Even if there is violence in his acts, he does not incur any good or bad fruits of his actions as his Karmas or acts become "akarma" or non-acts. This ultimately leads him to the state of peace or bliss.

Effect of Philosophy on Health

Philosophy of a person has a profound effect upon the health of a person. The correct philosophy not only acts as a shock absorber in life but also gives a person good health and peace of mind. Health has two components, that is, Physical Health and Mental Health. Before discussing the effect of philosophy on health, I would like to give a few tips for optimizing your physical and mental health.

1. Lead a simple and honest life keeping your requirements in life to the minimum.
2. Either be a vegetarian or a complete vegan. However, if you lead a vegetarian or vegan lifestyle, supplement your diet with Vitamin B_{12}. Also, get your blood level of Vitamin D checked up and in case of deficiency take adequate supplement under medical supervision.
3. Take supplement of Omega–3 fatty acids in form of DHA which is found in Algal Oil (Vegetarian source of fish oil) and ALA which is found in flax seeds, flax seed oil, walnuts, walnut oil, chia seeds, canola oil etc.
4. Your diet should have adequate amounts of proteins, carbohydrates, essential fatty acids, vitamins, minerals and it should normally consist of cereals, pulses, nuts, fruits, vegetables and sprouts. Limit your total calories from fat to twenty percent.

5. You should eat whole foods like brown rice, whole wheat, whole fruits, vegetables and fruits along with their skin, and completely avoid refined foods like table sugar, white rice, polished cereals and pulses, refined wheat flour etc. Also eat home cooked food as far as possible.
6. Eat organically grown foods which contain minimum amount of toxic substances like insecticides and pesticides.
7. Exercise everyday of your life. You should do aerobic exercises like walking, jogging, cycling etc. for a minimum of half an hour every day, followed by at least half an hour of strengthening, stretching and resistance training exercises like weights, Yoga, pilates etc.
8. Have adequate amount of sleep of about seven to nine hours every day, preferably at the same time.
9. Avoid too much exposure to electronic gadgets like television, internet, smart phones, mobile etc. and switch them off at least two hours before you sleep.
10. Eat your dinner at least two hours before you sleep.
11. Spend some time everyday on activities like meditation, social work, recreation and relaxation.

The above guidelines will have a very positive effect on your physical and mental health. Now I will discuss the effect of philosophy on your health. Without philosophy your body is like a rudderless boat, or like an aircraft without a pilot which is bound to crash. Philosophy of people can be broadly divided into three categories. The first is of the people who think positively about themselves, that they are immortal, everything, creator, preserver and destroyer of this Universe, very rich, influential, powerful, handsome, beautiful and so on. They also think that this Universe is nothing but a small part of their mind. Such type of people are extremely hard working, swift in their actions and have very high aims in life, but they also suffer from various psychological and health problems like anxiety, short temper, acidity, insomnia, substance abuse, restlessness and various other related health problems.

The second category of people is of those who think negatively about themselves, that they are mortal, insignificant, small, powerless, poor, illusory, nothing, temporary, ugly, weak and so on. They also think that they were not there before birth and would not be there after death, and therefore in between also they are nothing but an illusion. Such category of people have low aims in life, lack interest in various activities and are very slow. They also suffer from various psychological and health problems like depression, self-pity, sadism, panic attacks, stroke, heart disease, insomnia, substance abuse and related health problems.

Now, the third category of people is of those who take a balanced view of life and think that they are neither living nor dead, neither happy nor unhappy, neither good nor bad, neither superior nor inferior and so on, and base their thinking on philosophy that one side of duality like life–death, happiness–sorrow, good–evil, negative–positive and so on shall always be equal to the other side and one cannot exist without an equal amount of the other and therefore there is nothing to achieve or lose in this world.

Such types of people lead a balanced and healthy life and do all their duties in life without any attachment or aversion, and ultimately attain health, peace and bliss.

Henceforth, it can be concluded that philosophy has a profound effect upon the mental and physical health of a person and when it is combined with other guidelines as mentioned above, a person can lead a balanced, healthy and peaceful life.

Good and Bad Karmas

Everybody tells you to do good Karmas in life and keep away from bad Karmas, but the biggest problem is how to differentiate between good and bad Karmas, as every human action can be interpreted in two equal and opposite ways depending upon the time, place, person or circumstance under which it has been done. For example, let us start with time. A Karma at one point of time may be good Karma but the same Karma done at another point of time may be a bad Karma. There are innumerable examples under this category. Systems such as caste, slavery, blindly following various religious practices, discrimination on the basis of caste, color and religion, hunting wild animals and so on were considered good Karmas in the past, but are considered bad Karmas today. Similarly, there are many acts considered good Karmas today like engaging servants, drivers, and such other employees, which might be considered bad Karmas tomorrow, just like slavery is looked at today.

Now let us look at the place. Here, again you will find that a Karma considered good at one place or country might be a bad Karma at another place or country. There are innumerable examples in this categories also–equality and freedom of women in one country may be good Karma, but in another country it may be bad Karma, or providing information about the movement of army of the enemy country may be good Karma in that country, but a bad Karma in the enemy country, or supplying water in an area reeling under drought may be considered a good Karma, but supplying water to a flooded area may be a bad Karma.

Now let us look at a person or section of society, how a good Karma for one person or section of society might be a bad Karma for another person or section of society. In this category also examples are innumerable. A fighter may be regarded as a freedom fighter by one section but a terrorist by another, or religious freedom may be good Karma in one country but a bad Karma in another country, or feeding stray dogs, monkeys, snakes etc. or giving alms to beggars may be considered good Karma by one section of society, but a nuisance and bad Karma by another section of society.

Now let us look at the circumstances under which an act becomes good or bad Karma. There are innumerable examples in this category also, like a truth which is regarded as good Karma will become bad Karma if it leads to the killing of innocent people by passing on the correct information about their place of hiding to terrorists and dacoits. Similarly, consuming more calories during malnutrition may be a good Karma, but same during obesity may be a bad Karma. Similarly having a large number of children in an over populated and poor country may be a bad Karma, but in a rich and under populated country, it may be a good Karma.

From the above discussion it is clear that every human activity or karma has an equal amount of good and evil in it, and they cannot be separated out from each other. Apart from the examples already given above, there are innumerable other examples such as the building of dams, factories, agriculture, industrialization and so on. In the Bhagavad–Gita, Lord Krishna tells Arjuna that just as fire is always accompanied by smoke, similarly all human activities have some or the other negative aspect or vice (dosha) in them (chapter 18, verse 47).

Now the question is that if every human action has an equal amount of good and evil in it, then how should a person conduct himself, as no person can remain without work even for a moment? The answer is that the person should conduct himself in a manner which is acceptable to the society at that given point of time, place, circumstance or law, without any attachment or aversion to the results.

The person should try to meet all the reasonable expectations of the society in which he is living, without any desire or hatred. This can only be when he understands that there is nothing to achieve or lose in this world, as good and bad Karmas are also two sides of dualities like life–death, happiness–sorrow, gain–loss and so on, which are always equal to each other, and one cannot exist without an equal amount of the other.

The person who understands the above truth not only attains peace himself, but also spreads that peace in the society, while an ignorant person who classifies his Karmas either good or bad, not only remains disturbed and restless himself, but also spreads that restlessness and disturbance in the society in the form of anxiety, depression, anger, fear and so on.

Therefore, the person who sees good karma in bad karma and bad karma in good karma, like all other dualities like life–death, happiness–sorrow, gain–loss and so on, rises above these dualities and attains the ultimate peace and bliss.

Introduction to Vedanta

Vedanta means the end of the Vedas or the ultimate Knowledge of the Vedas. The said ultimate Knowledge refers to the Knowledge necessary for liberation of a person or for attaining the highest goal in life or God. The said Vedantas are also called 'Upanishads'. There are eleven main Upanishads, out of which I will briefly discuss the philosophy of nine Upanishads.

The first is 'Ishavasyopnishad' which is the 40th chapter of Shuklayajurveda. As the name suggests, the Upanishad explains God. It states that God is in everything and everything is in God, and whatever duties a person performs in life, should be done without any desire for fruits and for God only. It defines God as one, all pervading, faster than mind, indestructible, self illuminating, beyond injury, creator of everything, without any beginning or end and omnipotent. It states that the person who knows and worships Him also becomes immortal and unites with Him.

The second Upanishad is 'Kenopnishad' which is contained in Saamveda. This Upanishad explains God in a Question and Answer form between the student and the teacher. Here the teacher or Guru explains that God is mind of the mind, eye of the eye, ear of the ear and so on, and is beyond mind and senses. There is a story in it that once demi–gods defeated demons and falsely thought that they have won the battle due to their own efforts, due to their false ego. In order to teach them a lesson, God appears before them disguised as a Yaksha and proves that they are totally powerless before Him, and whatever victory they had was His blessings, and shattered their false ego. In the end this Upanishad states that the person who knows God becomes one with Him and merges in Him.

The third Upanishad is 'Kathopnishad' which contains the story of a child Nachiketa, who dies due to the curse of his father, and goes to the Demi God of Death or Yama, and asks him the question as to what happens to a person after he dies? Yama tries to bribe him with all the pleasures available on the earth and heaven in lieu of the question but fails. Then he explains to him that God or soul is indestructible, formless, endless, all pervading, self illuminating, hidden in the heart of all life forms and omnipotent. He explains that it is God or soul only that survives after the body dies and the person who knows the above truth rises above the dualities of pleasure and pain and becomes one with God. After giving him this knowledge he sent him back to earth.

The fourth Upanishad is 'Prashnopnishad' which is part of Atharvaveda. Here also six students go to a teacher or Guru and ask him questions about God. The teacher teaches them the importance of prana or breath, Om, and in the end teaches them about God, and states that He is indestructible and resides within all bodies along with the sixteen powers which are breath (prana), devotion, five basic elements (Earth, Water, Air, Fire, Sky), mind, senses, food, power to reproduce (Veerya), control of mind and senses (Tapa), various mantras, karma, different worlds (like heaven, earth, hell etc.) and their name. In the end he states that in the way that all rivers ultimately end in the ocean, similarly all these sixteen powers which came out of God, ultimately end in God, and the person who knows Him ultimately becomes one with Him and attains liberation.

The fifth Upanishad is 'Mundakopnishad' which is part of 'Atharvaveda'. It states that the creator of the Universe, Lord Brahma gave the ultimate Knowledge (Brahmvidya) to Atharva who passed it on to others. This Knowledge states that God is indestructible, formless, all pervading, Omnipotent, Omnipresent, beyond mind and senses, pure, higher than soul, nectar of immortality (Amrit), resides in the hearts of all living beings and is self illuminating. He is the creator and destroyer of the world, like a spider which creates its web from itself and swallows it. It states that God can only be attained through knowledge imparted by Guru and not by Karmas. In it God and soul have been compared with two birds who reside on a tree (human body), where soul enjoys the fruits of actions while God only looks on. The soul can be liberated only if it knows God and such knowledge of God destroys good and bad Karma, makes a person rise above dualities, become immortal and attain oneness with God.

The sixth Upanishad is 'Mandukyopnishad' which states that God has four legs. The first leg is a person with seven organs (various worlds) and nineteen faces (ten senses, five breaths, mind, ego, intelligence, nature) who experiences the real world. The second is again a person with seven organs and nineteen faces who experiences the dream world (during sleep). The third again is a person with seven organs and nineteen faces who experiences nothing during sleep. The fourth is the person who is formless, one, conscious, beyond mind and senses knowledge and is neither known nor unknown. The four legged God is represented by 'Om' which again has three legs which are actual world, dream world and sleep world. The formless Om is the above described fourth leg of the God who is the cause of the world, omnipotent, knows everything, is indestructible, and is creator, preserver and destroyer of this Universe. It is further stated that the person who knows God gets all the pleasures in this world, becomes all powerful, and ultimately merges in God and becomes one with Him.

The seventh Upanishad is 'Aitareyopnishad' which is part of Rigveda. It states that before this Universe came into existence, only God was there, Who decided to create this Universe and created it through His desire. Then He created a human body which was accepted by all the demi–gods he had created, and Himself also entered into it through head (Brahmarandhra). Then it describes three births of a man which are, first as his own son in the womb of his wife. The second is when he his born as a son outside the womb, and third when the person himself dies and is reborn. In the end it finally describes that the person who understands that he has been entrapped by millions of bodies in the past is liberated. It also states that the person who understands that God is immortal, everything, omnipresent, omnipotent, all powerful, pure knowledge and has manifested Himself in the form of this Universe, enjoys all the divine pleasure and merges in Him.

The eighth Upanishad 'Taittiriyopnishad', which is part of Yajurveda. This Upanishad teaches the method of worship, importance of 'Om', various duties of a person and good conduct. It states that a person has five bodies. The outermost body is made up of food (Anna), within which there are four more bodies which are made up of breath (Prana), mind (Mana), knowledge (Vigyan) and bliss (Ananda), respectively. It states that the person without desire enjoys the highest bliss in this Universe. It describes God as pure knowledge, everything, all powerful, indestructible, 'Om', self illuminating, residing in the cave of the hearts of all living beings, truth, bliss, omnipresent, omnipotent and creator, preserver and destroyer of this Universe. It states that the person who knows him becomes indestructible, blissful and merges in him.

The ninth Upanishad is 'Shwetashwataropnishad' which is named after a sage of the same name who meditated upon God and realized the ultimate truth. He describes God as indestructible, all encompassing, all powerful, endless, pure knowledge, one, knower of everything, 'Om', residing in the cave of the hearts of all living beings, formless, Omnipotent, Omnipresent, soul of all living beings, smaller than the smallest and bigger than the biggest, beyond mind and senses, beyond time, and witness of everything. He also teaches meditation and various powers that a Yogi can attain through it. In the end he says that the method to realize God is through the above knowledge, Karma Yoga and Gyan Yoga. The person who realizes Him destroys all his bondages, becomes indestructible and merges in Him.

From the above description it is clear that all the Upanishad teach us that a person should conquer all his desires, rise above the dualities and do his duties in life without any attachment or aversion to results.

A person can rise above dualities if he understands that there is nothing to achieve or lose in this world, as one side of duality like life–death, happiness–sorrow, good–evil, day–night and so on shall always be equal to each other, and one cannot exist without an equal amount of the other.

The person who understands the above truth becomes indifferent to all situations in life and a Karmayogi, and finally attains ultimate peace, bliss or God.

The Guru

There are certain fundamental questions that bother every person who has taken birth on this earth, such as, "Who am I? What is the purpose of my existence? Where was I before my birth? Where will I go after my death? What is true happiness? What is true knowledge?" and so on. Most people are unable to find answers and try to run away from these questions. Some of the common methods employed by them to avoid these questions are keeping themselves busy all the time in worldly activities, over socializing, reading books and using electronic gadgets like television, internet etc. only for the purpose of entertainment, travelling too much, drinking, substance abuse, etc. But there are certain people who are really interested and serious about finding the answers to their questions and try to look up various sources including an able person to guide them in life. The person who is really able to guide you in life is called as Guru or teacher. By Guru or teacher we do not mean the ordinary classroom teacher who provides you information about worldly affairs like business, politics, science etc., but a person who answers or guides you through the toughest and most fundamental questions of life as discussed above. Ancient Vedic philosophy has given great importance to "Guru" and has equated him to God. The various qualities of a true Guru as prescribed in Vedic philosophy are that he should be highly educated, detached, honest, risen above the dualities like happiness–sorrow, good–evil and so on, indifferent to various ups and downs in life, simple, dedicated, enlightened in mind, forgiving, keeps his mind and senses under control, knows answer to all the questions, is a man of few words, devoted, keeps his requirements in life to the bare minimum, does not keep any company, does not accumulate wealth and is contented with whatever he has.

Now a seeker who is seeking answer to these fundamental questions finds it extremely difficult to find such a person as mentioned above as such people or Gurus do not keep much company, maintain silence most of the time and refrain from displaying their knowledge as they have no desires, and understand that there is nothing to achieve or lose in this world. Even if with the blessings of God, one is able to find a true Guru, then also it is not necessary that he will be able to understand the meaning of the teachings of his Guru, as the capacity to understand differs from person to person depending upon their devotion, knowledge, experience, curiosity, intellectual capacity and so on. Also your own reasoning may not accept the teachings of the Guru. Ultimately, you will have to rely upon your own self to find out the answers to the above questions. Lord Krishna has at several places including Shrimad Bhagvat Purana (Para 11 Ch. 26 & 27) stated that "I am the ultimate Guru or teacher of every person and reside in the hearts of all living beings as their soul." Also, a person who is sensitive enough knows that there is a Guru in the heart of every person who guides that person from within all the time. This Guru has many names like conscience, inner voice, soul, God, Guru and so on.

A person can hear this Guru only if he is prepared to sacrifice anything in life to seek answers to his questions, including his own life, and follows certain practices like honesty, speaking only when necessary, eating nutritious and balanced food, keeping company only when necessary, forgiveness, meditation, cleanliness, control over mind and senses, pondering over the questions that he is seeking answers to, and giving up worldly desires and pleasures. Once the Guru within you is satisfied with your true intentions, he will take over and start guiding you. You will notice that all the answers that you are seeking in life are flowing out of the mouth of that Guru within you. If any person tries to suppress that voice of Guru, then that suppression is clearly visible in the form of disturbances and facial expressions, and the effort at over suppression leads to various diseases and sufferings. But the person who does not try to deceive himself, and listens to the voice of his Guru, and follows his instructions, becomes peaceful and contented from within when he gets all the answers to his questions. He soon rises above the dualities of life–death, happiness–sorrow, good–evil and so on, and understands that there is nothing to achieve or lose in this world, as the two sides of the dualities like life–death, good–evil, negative–positive and so on shall always be equal to each other, and one cannot exist without an equal amount of the other. This knowledge ultimately leads him to true peace and bliss.

Religion Versus Science

Religion refers to belief in and worship of God or a particular system of faith or worship while science refers to study or knowledge of the Physical and Natural world based on observations and experiments.

There is science in every religion and religion in every science. What was science yesterday is an outdated religion today, and what is science today may be an outdated religion tomorrow. Religion is the foundation on which the present day civilization stands. Without it, the entire building will collapse like a pack of cards.

It is true that science has provided us with all the comforts and luxuries, but it has also many negative aspects which are equal to its benefits. It has caused colossal damage to nature and environment that have taken billions of years to evolve and reach the present state of diversity.

Human beings with the help of science have already caused immense damage to marine life which has been reduced by half in the last 40 years. Similar damage has been caused to the animal kingdom, plant life and rainforests on the earth.

The damage to human life is no less, as millions of people die every year due to man–made pollution. Though the life span of people has improved, the quality of life has gone down. Earlier people used to enjoy nature, the trees, birds, sunset, rivers and oceans around them, but today you see only concrete jungles, pollution, honking of cars and diseases all around you. Everybody is in a great rush to make more money and increase the pollution further. Population of human beings is exploding and everywhere there is lack of natural resources like water, open spaces and clean air. Nations are sitting on a pile of nuclear weapons ready to annihilate each other at the slightest provocation, failing to understand that nuclear war even on a small scale is sufficient to wipe out the entire life on this planet.

The above discussion does not mean that religion is the cure of all the ills that we face today. Religion conferred many benefits on humanity; it provided people with peace of mind and oneness with nature. The human population was kept in check due to lack of the medical care that we have today. There was diversity, open spaces and greenery around us. People used to gather and celebrate various religious functions together. Everybody in the town knew each other, unlike as at present where even your neighbors don't know you. Everybody had a sense of purpose in life. It acted as a shock absorber in life, as whenever people faced adversity they had something to fall back upon, unlike today when people rush to chemists for mood altering drugs. Per capita consumption was much less due to lack of technology, and whatever was consumed by humans, nature was able to restore it. Though the life span was shorter, the quality of life was high which compensated for it.

Religion had its negative points also, such as it encouraged superstition and false beliefs. Though it united people practicing the same religion, it divided them against other religions. Any person who used to offend religious beliefs was punished disproportionately to his crime. There was lack of the present day comforts which are products of Science and Technology. People had to work hard to meet their daily needs though it also had a positive effect on their health. Proper medical care was not available and people mostly relied on traditional/herbal medicine which was ineffective in certain conditions, although it is also true that they suffered less from the side effects of medicine. Infectious diseases wiped out large portions of population. People were wholly dependent upon nature and used to face great hardship during floods and famine. Many people were regularly killed in man/animal conflicts and so on.

Now, the question arises that when both science and religion have their negative and positive aspects which are equal to each other, then how should we chose one over the other?

The answer is that both science and religion are equally important for us. If science provides us with present day comforts, religion provides us with moral support and a purpose in life. If science is best for removing our physical discomforts, then religion is best for removing our moral discomforts. We should try to exploit the positive aspects of both science and religion, and keep away from their negative aspects. On the one hand we should try to reduce our per capita consumption through vegetarian lifestyle, and by keeping our lives as simple as possible, and on the other hand we should devote more time to celebrate various religious functions and ceremonies with family and friends, and also devote more time on meditation. It has been scientifically proven that religious/spiritual people are more healthy and happy. To live your life to the fullest, a proper balance is to be maintained between science and religion after understanding that both are equally important aspects of our life.

There is science in every religion and religion in every science. They are both like inseparable twins which cannot be separated. In other words, they are two sides of the duality like life–death, happiness–sorrow, good–evil, day–night, and so on, where one side cannot exist without an equal amount of the other. The above understanding will lead to a purposeful balanced life, peace and harmony.

EFFECT OF KARMA ON FATE

Whenever something good or bad happens to us, we either blame it on our Karma or fate according to our convenience. But a deep analysis would show that both Karma and fate are equally responsible for whatever happens to us. For example, you are reading this article because of both your Karma as well as fate. It is your Karma as you desired to read an article on philosophy and made an effort in that direction, and it was your fate that this article was written by me and published on a particular date, time or place. Similarly, the people who argue that your Karma is solely responsible for whatever happens to you fail to understand that there are many people who want to do good or bad Karmas but are prevented by fate. For example, a child who wants to study very hard in life but is prevented from going to school/college due to poverty, or a criminal who wants to commit a crime but is prevented by heavy police presence in that area. Similarly, there are many people who hold fate to be responsible for what happens to them, who also fail to see that without Karma fate is no good. For example, a rich man may be having all the luxuries in life, still he will have to get up or move his hands and body to drink a glass of water, or a person who worked very hard day and night, but could not accomplish a task, while a person who worked very little was able to accomplish it. There are innumerable examples both in favor and against Karma and fate.

There are many people who say that your fate is nothing but the sum total of your past Karmas. They are also only partially correct as again your past Karmas also equally depended upon your fate as discussed above and vice versa.

If you try to examine this matter scientifically, then also you would find answers both in favor as well as against Karma and fate. For example, if we try to move an object from one place to another, then the force applied for that movement is our Karma but the gravity, resistance or tools available for that movement depends upon the fate. Another example, if you want to move an object to one kilometer on earth, you will need a particular force, while in space you can move that object to millions of kilometers with a fraction of that force. There are innumerable examples like the above.

Now, if we try to look at our ancient Vedic philosophy, there again we find conflicting answers. The entire religion is a code of conduct and it teaches a person how to conduct himself in a particular manner to attain heaven/liberation/peace/happiness. The ancient Vedic philosophy also states that no person can remain without Karma even for a moment and he should conduct himself in a particular manner to attain various objects in life. On the other hand, it also states that not even a blade of grass can move without the will of God and whatever happens on this earth is predestined or the will of God. Now the biggest question is that if everything is predestined and depends upon God, then why should we do any Karma at all, and if everything depends on our Karma, then where is the need for God or destiny? In other words, if everything either depends upon God or Karma, then either religion is useless or God does not exist. So if you go by religion, then also the answers would be conflicting.

Now, if we look at the law of the country, then also we find conflicting answers, as on one hand it has prescribed clear do's and don'ts and punishes or rewards the person who conducts himself in a particular manner, while on the other hand it talks about leniency, different set of punishments for same offence in different circumstances, reforms, mediation and remission of sentence in case of good conduct.

For example, when a person is killed by a criminal during a planned robbery, here the criminal gets a strict punishment, but when a person is killed by another man due to error of judgment or in self defense, here the person is acquitted. In other words, it also admits that circumstances or fate play an equally important role for determination of punishment or reward.

Now after getting disappointed from science, religion and law of the country, if a person sits down and analyzes his life and experiences to find out the answer, he will again be disappointed as on the one hand he will find that he was fully responsible for each and every action that he took in his life, on the other hand, he will find that he had nothing to do with it as everything depended upon circumstances, education, parents, experiences, religious beliefs, friends, economic conditions and innumerable other factors both within and outside his body. He will also observe that his body consists of trillions of microbes and cells and every thought that enters his mind or every decision that he takes might be a joint effort of all of them, and innumerable other factors both within and outside his body, and he may not have anything to do with it.

From the above discussion it is clear that both Karma and fate play equally important roles in your life. Now the biggest question is that once we understand the above truth how should we conduct ourselves?

The answer is that you should behave in a manner that you expect other people to behave with you, or in a manner that is acceptable to society and in conformity with the law of the land, without any attachment or aversion and leave its results to destiny/god/fate.

You can do so if you understand that Karma and fate are two sides of the dualities like life–death, good–evil, happiness–sorrow, day–night and so on, which shall always be equal to each other and one cannot exist without an equal amount of the other. The person who understands the above truth becomes detached and indifferent to the fruits of his actions and attains the highest state or perfect peace and bliss.

TIME

Whatever has been created shall be destroyed one day and whatever has been destroyed shall be recreated. This process of creation and destruction is a constant process like a wave which keeps on going up and down. The human mind is capable of calculating the rate at which this change is taking place. The said rate is called time. When we see the time vertically it is time, and when we look at it horizontally it is space. It is time/space that has separated the two sides of dualities like life–death, happiness–sorrow, good–evil, negative–positive and so on, which are always equal to each other, and derive their existence from each other. In other words, if time/space is not there, then this whole world would collapse into non-duality, that is, it will be neither alive nor dead, neither good nor evil, neither light nor darkness, neither day nor night and so on. It is the time/space that separates the two sides of duality from each other and rotates it like a wheel in such a manner that one follows the other. This process has been continuing endlessly. Time is relative, that is, it may differ according to person, object or situation. A billion years for you, may be a moment for somebody, and vice versa. Also, you may experience a life of hundred years in a dream lasting a few hours, or a hundred years of your real life may appear to you like a dream lasting a few hours.

Now the question is, who created this time and how did it come into existence?

The answer is that it is your own desires that have created the time. Earlier everything within you was in complete harmony, and you experienced a state of perfect peace and bliss as you were neither living nor dead, neither good nor evil, neither light nor darkness, neither happy nor unhappy, and so on. Then arose desire within you to experience something new. This desire assumed the form of time/space which separated out the dualities like life–death, good–evil, day–night and so on, which are always equal to each other, and follow each other, and started rotating them like a wheel or like a wave which keep on going up down, so that one follows the other in equal proportions. After they were separated out by time/space, you lost the harmony and became disturbed and started experiencing these dualities, that is, sometimes you experienced life and sometimes death, sometimes you were happy and sometimes unhappy, and so on. The greater your desires are, the more you experience these dualities. For example when you are very anxious about something, every moment appears to pass like years, and when you do not expect anything, then, the time just flies. In other words, this Universe of endless dualities expands with increase in your desires, and contracts with reduction in your desires.

It came into existence because of your desires. The more your desires increase, the more it expands. If your desires decrease, then this Universe also starts contracting. It can also come to an end with a big crunch or attain the state of non-duality, if you are able to attain the state of no desire or complete indifference.

Now the question is what is the root cause of desire? The root cause of desire is that you are not satisfied with what you have in the present and want to try something new. Then you start thinking about other possibilities and slowly and steadily you become one with them. You start feeling incomplete without those objects and make efforts to attain them. The more you obtain them, the more you want, like adding fuel to fire because you are running after a mirage. The only way to overcome such desires is to understand that if you cannot be satisfied with whatever you have today, you won't be in future also, irrespective of what you achieve. Whenever your mind tries to run after various objects of senses, you have to convince it that there is nothing to achieve or lose in this world, as one side of the duality shall always be equal to the other and one cannot exist without an equal amount of the other. Once you understand the above truth, your mind will settle down and time will slow down. Slowly and steadily, with practice, you will attain the state of no desire and complete indifference. Such an indifference would defeat the time and you will again attain your real state of non-duality and peace.

Karmayoga Versus Gyanyoga and Bhaktiyoga

In Matsya–purana (chapter 92), Lord Vishnu says that Karma Yoga is thousands of time more superior to Gyan Yoga, as knowledge or Gyana is a product of Karma Yoga, and therefore Karmayoga is the highest step (parama–pada). In the Bhagvad Gita also Lord Krishna clearly states that Karma Yoga is the highest form of Yoga (chapter 12, verse 11).

Before we discuss the importance of Karma Yoga, I would briefly explain the other forms of Yoga.

Lord Krishna in the Bhagvad Gita, has defined Yoga as 'Samatva' (chapter 2, verse 46) which means equanimity, equality and indifference. Similarly in Patanjali Yoga–sutra, Yoga has been defined as "Chittavratinirodha" which means control of mind, or preventing it from wandering in the pursuit of various object of senses, and attaining indifference towards the world.

Ancient Vedic philosophy has described many paths to Yoga which are stated below along with their drawbacks as compared to Karma Yoga.

1. **Mantra Yoga:** In Mantra Yoga, a mantra is given by the teacher to his disciple which is to be recited repeatedly along with following certain practices or 'Niyama' prescribed by the teacher, such as, non-violence, truth etc. The said practice destroys

sins, purifies the mind and prepares a person for higher forms of Yoga.

2. **Laya Yoga**: It refers to concentrating upon the void in the sky or the various sounds emanating from within the body like buzzing of hornets, musical notes on flutes, vibrations on Veena, ringing of bells and thunder clap. The said practice destroys sin, purifies the mind and prepares a person for the higher forms of Yoga.

3. **Hatha Yoga**: The said Yoga is concerned with the physical state of the body and makes it free from disease, decay and sins, and prepares a person for the next higher form of Yoga known as Raja Yoga. It prescribes various practices like abstinence, Asanas (postures), Pranayama (breath control) and Mudras (exercises). Hatha Yoga without Raja Yoga, and Raja Yoga without Hatha Yoga are stated to be useless.

4. **Raja Yoga**: It is a meditation upon various chakras (power centers) in the body known as Mooladhara, Manipura, Anahata, Visuddha, Ajnapura and Sahasrara. It is done to awaken dormant psychic power or Goddess Kundalini, which lies at the entrance of Brahmarandhra in Mooladhara Chakra, like a coiled serpent which is stated to give many supernormal power to the Yogis, and they ultimately lose the sense of duality and merge with the supreme. The said Yoga is inferior to Bhakti, Gyana and Karma Yoga as the Yogi here practices Yoga without realizing the purpose, and through use of force which may lead to certain physical and mental health problems like depression, panic attacks and so on if practiced over a long period of

time. After practicing this form of Yoga for some time the aspirant will be forced to move towards higher forms of Yoga i.e. Bhakti, Gyana and Karma Yoga.

5. **Bhakti Yoga or Dhyana Yoga:** It is a meditation upon God in the form of Krishna, Vishnu, Shiva etc, who is seated in the heart of a Yogi, and is continued till the aspirant loses the sense of duality and becomes one with God. The problem with this form of Yoga is that here everything is God. In other words, only God exists and everything else in an illusion including the person practicing it. The practice of this Yoga over a long period of time would expose the aspirant to various physical and psychological health problems like depression, panic attacks, low self–esteem, and insomnia. After practicing this form of Yoga for sometime, a person would be forced to move on to higher forms of Yoga, that is, Gyana and Karma Yoga.

6. **Gyana Yoga or Saankhya Yoga:** It refers to the knowledge of the entire Universe or self. This Yoga has subdivided the entire Universe including self into non–living and living, or nature (Prakriti) and soul (purush). It has further subdivided our body or nature (Prakriti) into twenty-four parts, which are invisible basic nature, intelligence, ego, mind, five basic elements, ten senses and five object of senses, and states that our body is destructible while we are the soul in this body which is indestructible, and also we are the creator, preserver and destroyer of this Universe. It has compared us or soul to a spider, and our body or Universe to its web, and states that as the spider

creates its web out of its own self, lives in it, and then swallows it, similarly we or soul also create this Universe/body out of ourselves, live in it, and ultimately destroy or swallow it. The problem with this Yoga is that it will lead you to a conclusion that you are everything and immortal, and everything else is an illusion which is incorrect, and will cause several physical and mental health problems like anxiety, hyper activity, acidity, insomnia and so on. After you practice this form of Yoga for some time, you will be forced to move on to the highest form of Yoga which is the Karma Yoga.

7. **Karma Yoga:** It refers to a person performing his duties in life without any attachment or expectation of results, with a sense of duty and for God only. It is stated that no person can remain without work on this earth even for a moment, and therefore he should perform all his acts without any attachment to result and for God only. This form of Yoga is the best and would lead to peace and harmony, and the highest form of good for the society and for mankind. But the question is why the Karma Yoga is the best? The answer is that as far as the first three forms of Yoga, that is, Mantra Yoga, Laya Yoga and Hatha Yoga are concerned, they are only means to the end, that is, they only prepare a person for higher forms of Yoga. As far as Raja Yoga is concerned it is inferior to Bhakti, Gyan and Karma Yoga as it is practiced by force without understanding the purpose, and would create health problems as already discussed and would ultimately push you towards higher forms of Yoga. As far as Bhakti Yoga and Gyana Yoga are

concerned, they are exactly opposite to each other, as in Bhakti Yoga you are nothing, while in Gyana Yoga, you are everything and immortal. Both would create health problems for you as discussed above and push you towards the middle path that is Karma Yoga, which is the highest form of Yoga, which will give you the benefits of all other forms of Yoga. All the other six forms of Yoga discussed earlier are like six steps of a staircase, which will lead you to the highest step (parama–pada), which is Karma Yoga.

The only problem with Karma Yoga is that scriptures have not properly explained as to why a person should not expect result or be attached to it, when every person in the world only works for some result or reward.

The answer is, because there is nothing to achieve or lose in this world, as the two sides, dualities like life–death, happiness–sorrow, good–evil, light–darkness and so on shall always be equal to each other, and one side cannot exist without an equal amount of the other. In other words, no situation in life is better or worse than the other.

The person who understands the above truth becomes a Karma Yogi and attains the highest form of peace or Samadhi.

THE COST OF SUCCESS

Everybody admires a person who is successful in life and hopes to reach that position one day. They see the positive side of success like name, fame, wealth, power, position etc. but fail to notice the cost the person has paid to reach that position. If you carefully analyze the cost that person has paid for success, you will find that it is always equal to the gains that he has made as a successful person. Similarly, the person who appears to be unsuccessful to us has also made certain gains in life which shall always be equal to his loss as a failed person. There are innumerable examples and some of them are discussed below.

First, let us take the case of Ramayana where Lord Rama successfully defeats and kills the demon Ravana. But if you carefully analyze the cost of that victory you will find that it was equivalent to his gains. First of all he was banished to the jungle for fourteen years. Then his beloved wife Sita was kidnapped by Ravana. After great effort and with the help of the army of monkeys and bears, he was able to defeat Ravana, and regain his wife and kingdom, but had to again banish her to a jungle, where she raised her two children. Afterwards, he also had to abandon his beloved brother Lakshmana, who went away and took Jal Samadhi in River Saryu. As a king also he lived a simple and disciplined life, did not remarry, and was extremely depressed. Hence, the cost that he paid for victory was equal to his gain in the victory. Similarly, Ravana also lost nothing as he attained Moksha (liberation) after he was again killed as "Sisupala" by Lord Krishna in his next rebirth, and attained the highest state or Moksha which is even envied by the greatest Yogis. Hence, his loss was also equal to his gain.

Now let us take the case of 'Mahabharata' where the 'Pandavas' defeated the 'Kauravas'. Here also, the cost of victory was extremely high as only six to seven persons survived the battle on both the sides, and nobody was left behind to enjoy the victory. Yudhishtira was extremely depressed after the victory, and cursed himself and his mother for all the destruction. Even after his death, he had to momentarily go to hell for lying to his Guru Dronacharya regarding the death of his son Ashwatthama. Similarly, even though the Kauravas lost the battle, they gained equally as they realized the highest desire of warriors of laying down their lives in the battlefield facing their enemy, and all of them went straight to heaven as their sins were washed out by the weapons with which they were killed.

Now, let us take the case of Lord Krishna. He had come to the earth to destroy all the demons who had taken birth as human beings and to reduce the burden of the earth. He fought many battles himself and through the Pandavas, and was successful in his purpose of eliminating all the demons from earth. But he had to pay a great price for it since his childhood. As a child his parents had to send him away to a forest, and they themselves were imprisoned by Kansa. Throughout his life he fought innumerable battles and before he left earth, all the male members of his entire clan (Yadavas), were destroyed due to internal feuds and the curse of Brahmins, though that was also his own will. Most of his over sixteen thousand wives were forced to either commit suicide by jumping into the river, or were kidnapped by dacoits who defeated Arjuna who was protecting them after Lord Krishna left the earth. His parents Devki and Vasudeva died out of the shock of losing their son. Only his one descendant Vajranabh, who was his great grandson, survived.

Similarly, the demons whom he killed also lost nothing, as they straight away went to heaven after their death as they were purified on being killed by the God Himself.

Now let us take the example of some great leaders of the world like Mahatma Gandhi and Nelson Mandela, who paid the cost of their success by remaining in jail for most of their lives. Similar is the case of Nobel peace prize winners, His Holiness the Dalai Lama who has lived as a refugee in India for most of his life, and MalalaYousafzai of Pakistan who was shot in the head and disfigured at a young age by the Taliban for fighting for the cause of education of girls.

Another is the case of the great scientist Stephen Hawking who is disabled neck downwards, and states that the reason for his success in life is his disability, as he was able to focus all his attention on scientific research because of it.

Also, if we take up the case of various wars fought by India, like the 1962 Indo-China War, where though India lost the war, a recent press report in the State controlled Chinese press states that China won nothing in the war except an enemy in its neighborhood, and the 1965 Indo-Pakistan war, where both the countries are equally celebrating their victories, shows that there are no losers or gainers in the war.

From the above examples we can conclude that every success in life comes with a cost which is equal to the gain, and vice versa. In other words, gain and loss are also two sides of dualities like life–death, happiness–sorrow, good–evil, day–night, negative–positive and so on which shall always be equal to the other, and one side cannot exist without an equal amount of the other.

The person who understands the above truth becomes a Yogi and attains the state of peace and harmony in life.

Body Versus Soul

Body of a person is defined as the physical structure of a person or animal, and the soul is defined as spiritual element of a person, believed by some to be immortal. As far as science is concerned, it does not distinguish between body and soul, and considers it to be one and the same. However, as far as ancient Vedic philosophy is concerned, the knowledge of the distinction between body and soul is considered to be the highest knowledge.

In chapter thirteen of the Bhagvad Gita, Lord Krishna explains the difference between Body and Soul to Arjuna. He subdivided the body into 24 parts or elements, which are unmanifested basic nature, intelligence, ego, five basic elements (earth, water, air, fire, sky), mind, ten senses (eyes, ears, nose, tongue, skin, voice, legs, hands, anus, genitals) and five objects of senses (smell, taste, form, touch, sound). He refers to body as 'Kshetra' (meaning area), destructible and 'Prakriti' (Nature). He defines soul as indestructible, all pervading, self illuminating, knowing, conscious and the one who experiences pleasure and pain etc. in the body. He refers to soul as 'Kshetragya' (knower of body), indestructible and 'Purush' (supreme God). From the above definition it is clear that the body is subject to birth and death, and does not have any consciousness, while the soul is immortal, conscious and experiences pleasure and pain in the body.

Now, the biggest question that has haunted mankind since time immemorial is whether we are the destructible body or the indestructible soul?

If we argue that we are only the body and different from the soul, then the biggest question that arises is that how can we experience pleasure and pain as the body does not have any consciousness or feeling. We should be like a stone which has no consciousness, feelings or emotion. It does not feel any pain or pleasure. It is incapable of taking any decision and is wholly dependent on the forces of nature. Therefore, the above assumption is not correct that we are the destructible body without any consciousness. The people who falsely believe that they are the destructible body, generally suffer from depression and lack of interest in life.

Now, if we argue that we are the indestructible, all pervading, self illuminating and conscious soul, then again the question arises that why is an indestructible soul trapped inside a destructible body? How can a small bird cage imprison something greater than a Sun? How can an inferior body hold or imprison a superior soul? Also, in case we are the indestructible soul, then why do we feel pleasure or pain which are related to body, or why do we sleep or become unconscious along with the body, and also why can't we leave it as per our own sweet will? Here, some people can argue that we are trapped inside this body because of the ignorance that we are the indestructible soul and the false belief that we are the body; then again the question will arise that how can an indestructible, self illuminating, all pervading soul be affected by ignorance, and why are many people who have obtained the knowledge that they are the indestructible soul, still trapped inside the body, and struggling hard to earn a living? Also, if we are the indestructible soul, then why don't we remember our past before we came into this body, and why don't we know where we will go after our body dies?

From the above discussion it is clear that we are not the indestructible soul either. People who falsely believe that they are the indestructible soul, generally suffer from anxiety, hyperactivity and acidity etc.

Now the question is that if we are neither the body nor the soul, then what are we?

The answer is that we are a product of both of them. We have equal amount of both body and soul in us. In other words, neither can we exist without a body, nor can we exist without a soul. This Body–Soul can be compared with Radha–Krishna or Shakti–Shiva. This body and soul are also two sides of a duality like life–death, happiness–sorrow, good–evil, day–night, positive–negative and so on, where one side cannot exist without an equal amount of the other. In other words, we are neither living nor dead, neither happy nor unhappy, neither good nor evil, neither body nor soul, neither positive nor negative, and so on, as one side of the duality shall always be equal to the other. The person who understands the above truth rises above these dualities and becomes detached and indifferent to all situations in life, and attains true peace and harmony in life.

Dreams Versus Reality

Since my childhood, whenever I see a dream at night, I get fascinated by it and think about the difference between the dream world and the real world. When we sit down and try to compare the two, we find that there is very little difference between the two as both are temporary, both follow a certain set of rules, and both are experienced by the same person. First of all, if we look at the temporary nature, then we find that just as dream is limited by time, our real life and this Universe are also limited by time; that is, both will come to an end one day. If we look at the set of rules to be followed, then also we find that in the way that various rules and regulations govern our lives in the real world, the same rules and regulations also apply to our dream world. Thirdly, if we look at the person experiencing it, then also we find it is the same person who is experiencing them both. The only difference between the two is of duration, that is, dream is of a shorter duration, while real life is of a longer duration. But this difference is also illusory, as time is relative and a person can experience a life of hundred years in a dream lasting a few hours, and hundred years of real life can appear to a person like a dream lasting for a few hours.

From the above discussion it is clear that there is no difference between the two, that is, the real world is as much an illusion as a dream world, and the dream world is as much a truth as the real world. Once this truth sinks into our mind, we suddenly feel detached from the real world, and start wondering whether all the efforts that we are making for our career, survival, family and so on are really worth it; that is, if the real world, is also like a dream, then why should we work so hard in life? As soon as you start thinking about the above question, you start moving in the right direction. That is, a person should do his duties in the world because it is half truth, and the person should be detached to the results because it is half illusion. In your dream also you see that you are working very hard to realize certain goals and objectives, but realize that it is meaningless only when you wake up from the sleep. Similarly, a wise person also thinks about the endless lives and deaths that he has experienced in the past, and understands the meaninglessness of all the efforts, attachments, Karmas, and emotions that we make or experience in life. Now, the question arises that if everything is meaningless, then why should we make an effort, and why should we not leave everything to fate or God? The answer is given in the Bhagvad Gita where Lord Krishna tells Arjun that no person in this Universe can remain without work even for a moment, and therefore he should perform his duties without any attachment to results. Now, if we analyze this statement, we find that there is an absolute truth in this statement, as giving up all activities means giving up even breathing. In order to live we have to breathe, drink water, eat food, protect ourselves from harmful organisms/animals/nature, socialize and take care of our family. Even if you give up all your work and jobs, you will find that you are working even harder than before, and it is much easier to lead a normal life and work for your living, than sitting idle at home. Even in your dream you work hard in order to survive, as whatever you do in your dream also affects your health and life. For example, when you see a nightmare, your heart beats much faster than in real life and vice visa.

The work that you do in your dream may be as important as the work that you do in the real world, for your survival. It is a scientific fact that without sleep we will not survive, as the body repairs itself, consolidates all its memories and rejuvenates itself during sleep, and dreaming may be a part of this process.

From the above discussion it is clear that life cannot exist without dreams and dreams cannot exist without life, and reality and illusion are also two sides of dualities like life–death, happiness–sorrow, good–evil, day–night and so on, where one side cannot exist without an equal amount of the other. The person who realizes the above truth becomes a Karmayogi and does all his duties without attachment or aversion to results, and attains peace, harmony and bliss.

DETACHMENT AND INDIFFERENCE

There is no end to human desire. The entire wealth in the Universe is not sufficient to satisfy even one person. The more a person tries to run after them, the more they increase like adding fuel to fire. Human beings are attached to many things in life like family, friends, wealth, fame, food and so on. The attachment comes when a person desires or starts thinking about an object of senses. Soon he forgets himself and becomes one with it, and starts identifying himself with that object.

He starts thinking that he is incomplete without that object. Even a thought of losing that object causes great pain in his heart. He forgets that whatever has been created in this world will come to an end one day including his own body, and whatever has been destroyed shall be re created. He is sitting on a swing of life which is moving to and fro, that is from creation to destruction, and destruction to creation. Every time he moves from creation to destruction he feels very sad, depressed and unhappy, and when he moves from destruction to creation he starts jumping with joy, and feels very excited and happy. People and objects of senses keep on meeting and leaving him like various twigs flowing in a river. All his problems arise because he differentiates between various objects as good–bad, friend–enemy and so on, but forgets that everything is the same. For example, various objects made from gold such as bracelet, earrings, necklace etc. are nothing but gold only. Similarly all the matter in this Universe is made up of the same atoms, the only difference being in its arrangement. There is unity in diversity and diversity in unity. The person runs after objects of senses like family, food, wealth, etc., thinking that they will give him more pleasure and happiness than himself, or than what he already has, but is disappointed. The temporary satisfaction or happiness that he gets from that object ultimately ends in an equal amount of dissatisfaction and unhappiness, and he soon realizes that he was running after a mirage. He forgets that even his own body for which he is making all the effort will come to an end one day, and everything would be left behind. He has come empty handed into this world, and would leave empty handed. He is all the time restlessly moving up and down between dualities like life–death, happiness–sorrow and so on like a wave.

The only way to rest in peace is to understand that every person in this world is born with a zero bank balance. The more he overdraws from that bank in the form of pleasure and happiness, the more he will have to pay back in the form of displeasure and unhappiness. The more he will deposit in it in the form of hard work and sacrifice, the more he will get back in the form of wealth and rewards. Ultimately, his bank balance would remain zero. In other words, the two sides of dualities in this world like life–death, happiness–sorrow, gain–loss, good–evil and so on shall always be equal to each other, and one cannot exist without an equal amount of the other. The person who understands the above truth knows that there is nothing to gain or lose in this world, and becomes detached and indifferent to all ups and downs of life, and attains the state of peace, harmony and bliss.

LOGIC BEHIND FORGIVENESS

There is no other friend or enemy in this world except one's own self. The person who searches for the truth and rises above the dualities, is his own friend, and an ignorant person who is torn between the dualities is his own enemy.

Forgiveness is the most discussed topic in various spiritual articles and occupies huge space in the philosophy of various religions.

Most of the articles on spirituality and religious books tell you about the importance of forgiveness but fail to explain to you the logic behind forgiveness and how to forgive. Because of lack of such knowledge we try to force ourselves physically to forgive a person, but keep on burning from inside with a desire to take revenge, which is another form of violence. The logic behind forgiveness is that no person in this world is either capable of harming you or giving you anything. Similarly, neither can you harm any person in life or give anything to anybody. It is all a matter of perception or it is only your mind which is creating the distinction of enemy and friend, or harm and gain. Every human act has an equal amount of good and evil in it. For example, giving alms to a beggar may be an act of charity or goodness as per your perception, but a big nuisance for your neighbors and society as a whole, and it is not surprising that the Government discourages such acts through anti beggary laws. Similarly, you may perceive that feeding monkeys or stray dogs is an act of kindness for you, but your neighbors might be abusing you for causing a big nuisance for them. Most of the successful people in this world give the credit for the success in their lives to the adversities or sufferings that they have faced at the hands of nature and other fellow human beings. When somebody abuses or harms you, he also gives you an opportunity to introspect and search for your shortcomings, which makes you a better and stronger person as you try to overcome those weaknesses. Also, you realize in the process that your actions in the past also caused similar pain to other people which you did not realize at that time, and you become a better human being. Therefore the act of harming you also equally benefits you. Even if you falsely believe that a person is capable of harming somebody, then also you will notice that when a person prepares for the act of harming another person, he first causes equal amount of harm to himself. For example, a person who slaps another person, first causes a pain equivalent to slapping upon himself and then slaps the other person. He has already given himself punishment for that act and there is no point in punishing him again. Similarly if you slap him back, you also first slap yourself and then hit him. Therefore, if you take revenge, you get two slaps instead of one. I once read an interview of a police officer who was an encounter specialist, who said that it caused him great pain, and took him several days to mentally prepare himself for an encounter with and killing of a dreaded criminal. Similarly, I know many judges who used to remain extremely disturbed for several days before they sentenced a dreaded criminal with death or life imprisonment, and prayed to God that they don't have to pronounce such a sentence again. Now, an important question is that when nobody is capable of harming anybody, or if a person has already given himself an equivalent punishment for causing pain to somebody, then why should the police catch a criminal, or judges punish them, or a soldier kill an enemy on the border.

The answer is that this act is necessary not for punishing the criminal, but for restraining other people from following a similar wrong behavior, as everybody does not understand the truth as stated above and starts thinking that doing wrong to other people is advantageous, and does not have any repercussions or demerits. As it is human nature to ape each other, if a criminal is not punished by law, then others, without realizing that he has already undergone punishment, start aping him, seeing only the merits of his crime. Therefore, if any person is entrusted with responsibility as police officer, judge or army officer, he should just do his duty without any desire or hatred, and only with a view of setting an example for others, and to prevent future repetition of such acts.

From the above discussion it is clear that there is no point in taking revenge, as every human act has an equal amount of good and evil in it, and good and evil are also two sides of the dualities like life–death, gain–loss, day–night, punishment–reward and so on, which shall always be equal to each other, and one cannot exist without an equal amount of the other.

The person who understands the above truth forgives everybody from within, rises above the dualities and attains ultimate peace and bliss.

Meditation

Before you start meditation, I would like to give certain tips which are beneficial for optimizing the results of Meditation:

1. Lead a vegetarian and simple life.
2. Take adequate sleep of 6–8 hours every day, preferably at the same time.
3. Exercise every day of your life with at least half an hour of aerobic exercises like walking, jogging, cycling etc, followed by at least half an hour of stretching, strengthening and resistance training exercises like Yoga, weight training, pilates etc.
4. Keep away from too much exposure to electronic gadgets like T.V., internet, mobile etc. and switch them off at least two hours before you sleep.
5. If you are a vegetarian or pure vegan, then get yourself checked for deficiency of Vitamins B_{12}, D and E, and in case you are deficient, take adequate supplements under medical supervision as these vitamins are essential for the proper functioning of your nervous system. Also, take supplements of Omega–3 fatty acids available in Algal oil (vegetarian sources of DHA–Fish oil), Flax seeds/ flax seed oil, walnut/walnut oil, chia seeds etc., as it is very beneficial for the health of your nervous system.

6. Lead a simple and honest life and also devote some time for social work.

The above tips are not essential for meditation but are beneficial for optimizing its results.

Now, certain things to be remembered before you begin meditation are:

1. Never force your mind into concentration or to attain any state. Meditation should only be done through convincing your mind with the truth, through auto suggestions.
2. Though meditation can be done anywhere or anytime, however it is advisable that you select a clean place or room with a peaceful atmosphere and little distraction. The surface on which you meditate should neither be too soft, nor too hard, with a preferable softness of about four fold woolen blanket.
3. You can meditate by either sitting on a chair or cross legged on any other surface. Your back and neck should be upright but relaxed. You can also lie down on your back in Shava–Asana.
4. Though any amount of meditation is beneficial, you can start with half an hour everyday and increase the time according to your comfort level. In case you feel uneasy at any time discontinue the same.

Now, sit down quietly, close your eyes and watch your mind for some time. You will find that your mind is restlessly wandering in the past or the future, and in search of various objects of senses for achieving certain goals in life, which you falsely believe will give you more happiness/

satisfaction than the present. Your mind is always running after endless desires under the false impression that their realization would give you more happiness than what you already have. The more it realizes those desires, the more they increase, like adding fuel to fire and the mind gets even more restless.

Now, make a suggestion to yourself there is nothing to gain or lose in this world, as the two sides of dualities like gain–loss, life–death, happiness–sorrow, good–evil, and so on shall always be equal to each other, and no situation in life is better or worse than the other. Keep on repeating this suggestion to yourself at regular intervals. After some time you will find that once your mind realizes the above truth, it has slowed down and has became more peaceful. Instead of running in the past or future, it has settled down in the present. Instead of moving out towards various objects of senses, it has moved inwards. With regular practice you will see that your sight will get fixed between your eyebrows. You will experience that time has slowed down and everything around you including your thoughts are moving in slow motion. You will also experience that your entire body has become illuminated and a bright white light is coming out of it, and it was you yourself whom you were searching for all the time. You will also experience divine emotions, music, objects, situations and beauty which are beyond words. Just watch all these experiences, without attachment or repulsion, and keep on reminding yourself at regular intervals that there is nothing to achieve or lose in this world, as your gain and loss shall always be equal in all situations, till you achieve the state of perfect peace, bliss or Samadhi.

The Three Brothers

Once upon a time there was a wise and learned Brahmin who earned his living by teaching students. He had three sons. His wife died immediately after giving birth to his youngest son and he did not remarry. He raised all his sons himself and taught them all the knowledge necessary for living a noble and honest life. All his three sons were also very dedicated and noble. His eldest son always used to think positively in life, so his father named him Gyana. His middle son always used to look at the negative aspects of life and he was named Dhyana by his father, and the youngest was neutral and took a balanced view of life, and was named Karma by the father. After imparting all the education to his sons, the father died and as he was very honest and a charitable person, he did not leave behind much wealth.

His younger brother resided in Rampur village, and made an offer to the three brothers that he would help them to set up a business if they came to his village, to which they readily agreed as they had no other source of income. The distance was long and there was no other transport, so they set out on foot along with some food and money that their father had left behind. While travelling, they had to cross a jungle. When they were in the middle of the jungle, they were attacked by a pack of stray dogs. On seeing the dogs charging towards them, Dhyana who always thought negatively, surrendered before those dogs, thinking that he is very weak and powerless, and one day he will die anyway.

The dogs badly mauled him. In the meantime, Gyana, who always thought positively in life, thought that he is very strong and powerful, and nobody in the world can kill or defeat him, attacked those dogs with his bare hands. When the dogs saw him charging towards them, they left his brother and badly mauled him also. In the meantime, Karma who always took a balanced view in life, thought that after a lot of good Karmas and good fortune, God has given me this human body and I should make all efforts to protect it and also save my brothers. Thinking thus, he quickly climbed a mango tree nearby, plucked some raw mangoes and started shouting and throwing those mangoes at the dogs. This diverted the attention of those dogs and they left Gyana and surrounded the tree where Karma was sitting, fiercely barking at him, and waited for him to come down. After some time they got tired and left. Karma came down the tree, collected some medicinal herbs and applied them on the wounds of his brothers. Soon his brothers recovered from the injuries and they reached a village on their way. As the three brothers were resting under a tree, the villagers suddenly started shouting that some dacoits are coming and asked everybody to hide. It was a small village and the villagers on hearing the warning quickly collected their valuables and hid themselves in the big house in the village. Some villagers also asked the three brothers to do the same but the older two refused and only Karma went along with them. Both the brothers thought that they have nothing with them, so what will the dacoits gain by harming them? The dacoits came and searched for the villagers but could not find them or the valuables, and saw the two brothers under the tree. They caught both of them and searched them but could not find anything. Then they caught hold of Dhyana and asked him about the place where the villagers were hiding. Dhyana again took a negative view and thought that one day he is going to die anyway, so why should he harm innocent villagers and incur sin for it? He also thought that he is very weak and powerless and no match for the dacoits, and therefore meekly surrendered before them, but clearly refused to give them the information. The dacoits got very angry and thrashed him badly. Then they asked Gyana about the villagers. Gyana again took a positive view that he is very strong and powerful and nobody can defeat or kill him. He then charged towards the dacoits but was caught by them and badly thrashed like his brother. Karma was watching all this helplessly and wanted to help his brothers, but took a balanced view that if he remains alive, only then he would be able to help himself and the injured brothers. He therefore remained in hiding. After the dacoits left empty handed, he again went to the jungle and collected medicinal herbs for his brothers and applied them on their wounds. Soon they recovered and the entire village thanked the brothers for not disclosing their hideout, and requested them to stay with them for some time. After staying with the villagers for a few days, they left for Rampur along with food and small gifts that the villagers gave them. After a few days they reached Rampur and their uncle fulfilled his promise and helped all the three in setting up their own small business. Gyana, the eldest brother again thought positively that he is very intelligent, hard working, immortal and powerful, and worked very hard day and night, and soon accumulated huge wealth. But in the process he also made a large number of enemies as he was extremely short tempered and a miser. Dhyana again took a negative view of life and thought that what is the use of all this when one day everything including my body would be reduced to dust? He also thought that he was very weak, stupid and powerless, and lost all his interest in the work. He used to pity himself and started incurring huge losses. Soon his business was shut down and he became totally dependent upon alms and the charity of other people. People used to abuse and humiliate him all the time, which he tolerated without any complaint. Now, the third brother Karma again took a balanced and moderate view of life and worked sufficiently hard to earn a living for a comfortable life. Whatever surplus he earned, he used to spend on charity including his elder brother Dhyana. After the three brothers had spent a few years in the village, there was a famine in the village due to drought. People soon started dying of hunger. With great difficulty, Karma took care of himself and Dhyana. However, Gyana was very comfortable as he had huge wealth. Seeing him comfortable, soon his enemies, competitors, employees whom he had humiliated due to his short temper and other villagers united against him due to jealousy, and attacked him. They looted all his wealth and left him badly injured. Karma had made a lot of friends in the village due to his charitable nature and pacified them against his brothers. After that he again took care of them and they soon recovered. One day, all the three sat down under a tree and started discussing about their past life and future course of action. Their father was a very noble person and had given them very good education in life. After a long discussion they reached the conclusion that they had wasted enough of their lives in pursuing materialistic pleasures, but did not find any peace or happiness, and now without wasting any more time, they should search for the ultimate truth, peace, bliss and God. After taking the above decision they left for a jungle with some food towards an Ashram of some wise Yogis. They went to them and started serving them as servants. After some time the Yogis were pleased with them and asked them what they wanted. The three brothers told them the purpose for which they had come to them and requested them to help them. The Yogis told them that every evening they used to sit down and discuss about the ultimate truth, peace, bliss and God, and the various methods to attain these, and the brothers should quietly sit down and listen to them. Every day the wise Yogis sat down and discussed about various forms of Yoga like Gyana Yoga, Bhakti Yoga, Karma Yoga, Raja Yoga etc., and the brothers soon learned all they wanted. They then left the Ashram after thanking and taking permission from the wise Yogis. After travelling for some time the brothers found a peaceful and quiet place in the jungle, and constructed an Ashram for pursuing their objective. The wise Yogis had taught them all the forms of Yoga or methods for achieving their objectives, and they had to select one of them that suited them the best. Again, according to their nature, Gyana selected Gyana Yoga which states that the person is himself an indestructible soul or God, and is creator, preserver and destroyer of this Universe, like a spider which creates its web from itself, lives in it and ultimately swallows it. He used to sit down and meditate all the time on this knowledge. Thinking himself to be immortal and all powerful, he soon gave up all activities in life and used to survive on whatever Karma gave him to eat or drink. Soon he became very weak and instead of achieving his objective of ultimate peace, bliss and God, he started suffering from severe anxiety and related health problems. Similarly, Dhayna, according to his nature selected Bhakti or Dhyana Yoga which states that everything is God, who is sitting in the lotus of the heart of every person, and a person should meditate upon him. He also started meditating upon this knowledge and gave up all the activities as he thought that if everything is God, then I am only an illusion and would come to an end one day, and then what is the use of all the efforts that I make in life? He also became very weak, and instead of achieving his objective he suffered from severe depression, panic attacks and related health problems. He also survived on whatever Karma gave him to eat or drink. Karma also, according to his nature selected Karma Yoga which states that a person should perform all his duties in life without any attachment or aversion to the fruits of his action and for God only. In other words, a person should perform all his duties in life efficiently and diligently, and leave the results to fate or God. Accordingly Karma used to lead a balanced life, taking care of all the necessities of life, and used to meditate in whatever time remained after performing his duties including looking after his brothers. Soon, he realized the purpose for which he had come to the jungle and his face started glowing with peace, bliss and knowledge. On seeing him, his brothers realized their mistake and asked him the secret of his success, to which he readily agreed.

They soon realized that they had been wrong throughout their lives by taking an unbalanced or extreme view, and followed the balanced middle path of Karma Yoga as shown by Karma, and soon realized their objective in life.

The three brothers represent the three types of personalities on this earth (i.e. optimistic, pessimistic and balanced), and the paths followed by them represent the three forms of Yoga, that is, Gyana Yoga, Bhakti Yoga and Karma Yoga.

To lead a balanced life it is necessary to understand that the two sides of dualities like life–death, good–evil, happiness–sorrow and so on, shall always be equal to each other, and one cannot exist without an equal amount of the other. The person who understands the above truth knows that there is nothing to achieve or lose in this world, and becomes a Karma Yogi and attains ultimate peace, bliss and God.